The E Renal Diet Cookbook

A Beginner's Guide With Low Sodium, Low Potassium & Low Phosphorus Recipes To Managing Kidney Disease And Avoiding Dialysis

Jodie Paige

derived from various sources. Please consult a licensed professional before attempting any techniques outlined in this book.

By reading this document, the reader agrees that under no circumstances is the author responsible for any losses, direct or indirect, which are incurred as a result of the use of information contained within this document, including, but not limited to, errors, omissions, or inaccuracies.

Table of Content

BREAKFAST 9

APPLE SAUCE CREAM TOAST 10

WAFFLES 11

EGG WHITES AND VEGGIE BAKE 13

PEACH BERRY PARFAIT 15

OPEN-FACED BAGEL BREAKFAST SANDWICH 16

OPEN BREAD WITH ALMOND 17

BIRCHER MUESLI WITH PAPAYA 18

CAULIFLOWER AND BROCCOLI CURRY 20

BROCCOLI AND LENTIL SALAD WITH MACKEREL 21

BROCCOLI RICE GRATIN (ITALIAN STYLE) 23

PINEAPPLE SMOOTHIE 25

EGG WHITE AND PEPPER OMELET 26

ITALIAN APPLE FRITTERS 27

TOFU AND MUSHROOM SCRAMBLE 29

EGG FRIED RICE 30

SIMPLE ZUCCHINI BBQ 32

LUNCH 35

SPICY CHICKPEAS WITH ROASTED VEGETABLES 36

SPECIAL VEGETABLE KITCHREE 38

MASHED SWEET POTATO BURRITOS 40

CHICKPEA SHAWARMA DIP 42

LIGHT MUSHROOM RISOTTO 44

VEGETABLE PIE 46

PURE DELISH SPINACH SALAD 48

SEXY SALSA SALAD 49

JALAPENO SALSA 50

CREAMY & CULTURE TOMATO SAUCE 51

WHITE VELVET CAULIFLOWER SOUP 53

RUSSIAN CABBAGE SOUP (SHCHI) 55

FENNEL AND PEAR SOUP 57

DINNER 60

ZUCCHINI AND TURKEY BURGER WITH JALAPENO PEPPERS 61

GNOCCHI AND CHICKEN DUMPLINGS 63

CREAMY TURKEY 65

LEMON PEPPER CHICKEN LEGS 67

POULTRY..**70**

ROASTED CARROT SOUP 71
GARLIC AND BUTTER-FLAVORED COD 73
TILAPIA BROCCOLI PLATTER.................................. 75
VERY WILD MUSHROOM PILAF 77
SPORTY BABY CARROTS 78
SAUCY GARLIC GREENS 80
SPICY HERB SEASONING 82
PHOSPHORUS-FREE BAKING POWDER...................... 83
BASIL OIL 84

SNACK **86**

.... 86
TOASTED PUMPKIN SEEDS..................................... 87
TOFU PUDDING 88
CHIA CASHEW CREAM 90
DRIED DATES & TURMERIC TRUFFLES...................... 91
COCO CHERRY BAKE-LESS BARS.............................. 92

DESSERT **94**

LEMON MOUSSE.. 95
JALAPENO CRISP 96
RASPBERRY POPSICLE... 98
EASY FUDGE 99

Breakfast

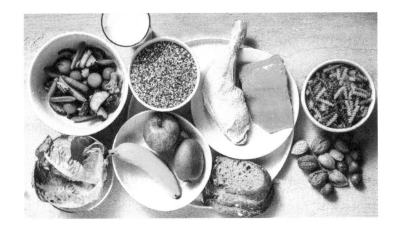

Apple Sauce Cream Toast

Preparation Time: 5 minutes

Cooking Time: 10 Minutes

Servings: 1

Ingredients:

- 2 tablespoons applesauce
- 2 slices of toast or white bread
- 1 egg white – uncooked, scrambled
- Cinnamon

Direction:

1. Whip the liquid uncooked egg white until foamy and take a skillet that doesn't stick. Heat the skillet then soak one side of the toast into the egg white whip.

2. Bake the toast on the side where the toast is soaked into the egg white and while you are doing so, soak another piece of toast into the egg white whip and as you are baking the second toast piece and applesauce on the second piece and seal with the first piece of toast once the outside crust is well baked.

3. Sprinkle with cinnamon to taste and serve.

Nutrition: Potassium 294 mg Sodium 366 mg Phosphorus 158 mg Calories 256

Waffles

Preparation Time: 20 minutes

Cooking Time: 15 Minutes

Servings: 8

Ingredients:

- 1 and ½ teaspoons yeast for baking
- 8 tablespoons butter – unsalted
- 2 eggs
- 1 and ¾ cups of milk – 2% milkfat
- Sugar substitute to taste
- 1 teaspoon almond extract
- 2 cups flour – all-purpose

Direction:

1.   Heat a saucepan and place the butter and milk in it. Wait for the butter to melt with occasional stirring. As you are waiting for the milk and butter mixture to cool off a bit so that the saucepan is warm to touch, you will take a bowl and whisk sugar substitute, yeast and flour. Once combined, you will add the warm milk and butter mixture to the flour bowl and whisk some more until the mass is well combined.

2.   Take another bowl and whisk the eggs with almond extract, adding the flour batter's whipped egg mixture. Stir in well to combine until you get a smooth, homogenous mass. The best option is to prepare the mixture a day ahead as you will need to keep the dough in the fridge for at least 12 hours before baking.

3.   Once you are ready to bake your waffles, you will set the oven to 200 degrees F and keep the waffle bowl near so that the dough is kept warm. Prepare your waffle maker and start making waffles by pouring the dough.

Nutrition: Potassium 131 mg Sodium 208 mg Phosphorus 113 mg Calories 223

Egg Whites and Veggie Bake

Preparation Time: 20 minutes

Cooking Time: 50 Minutes

Servings: 4

Ingredients:

- 1 cup broccoli florets
- 1 cup cauliflower florets
- 1 garlic clove - minced
- 6 egg whites – liquid, uncooked
- ½ cup bell pepper – diced
- 1 small onion – finely diced
- ½ cup low-sodium cheese

Direction:

1. Take care of the veggies, wash and dice the cauliflower, broccoli and onion. While you are sautéing onion with a tablespoon of olive oil, place broccoli and cauliflower in a bowl with a tablespoon water and place the bowl in the microwave.

2. Microwave florets for 5 minutes before taking the bowl out of the microwave. The onions should be ready within 5 minutes, when you should add the minced garlic and peppers. Sauté for another 3 to 4 minutes.

3. Combine broccoli and cauliflower florets with garlic, peppers and onion and let the veggie mixture cool off a bit as you are whisking egg whites. Egg whites should be whisked until foamy. Whisk in the cheese with the egg whites then add

the veggie mixture to your egg whites, stirring the ingredients to combine it into a homogenous mass.

4.   Take a medium baking dish and pour in the mixture. Preheat the oven to 350 degrees F and place the baking dish into the oven, baking the egg white veggie bake for 20 minutes or until the mixture settles.

Nutrition: Potassium 163 mg Sodium 89 mg Phosphorus 105 mg Calories 258

Peach Berry Parfait

Preparation Time: 5 minutes

Cooking Time: 5 minutes

Servings: 2 servings

Ingredients:

- 1 cup plain, unsweetened yogurt, divided
- 1 teaspoon vanilla extract
- 1 small peach, diced
- ½ cup blueberries
- 2 tablespoons walnut pieces

Directions:

1. In a small bowl, combine the yogurt and vanilla.

2. Put 2 tablespoons of yogurt to each of 2 cups. Divide the diced peach and the blueberries between the cups, and top with the remaining yogurt.

3. Sprinkle each cup with 1 tablespoon of walnut pieces.

Nutrition: Calories: 191; Total Fat: 10g; Saturated Fat: 3g; Cholesterol: 15mg; Carbohydrates: 14g; Fiber: 14g; Protein: 12g; Phosphorus: 189mg; Potassium: 327mg; Sodium: 40mg

Open-Faced Bagel Breakfast Sandwich

Preparation Time: 5 minutes

Cooking Time: 5 minutes

Servings: 2 servings

Ingredients:

- 1 multigrain bagel, halved
- 2 slices tomato
- 1 slice red onion
- Freshly ground black pepper
- 1 cup microgreens

Directions:

1. Lightly toast the bagel.

2. Place the bagel halves, top each half with 1 slice of tomato and a coupleof onion ringsn.

3. Season with the black pepper. Top each half with ½ cup of microgreens and serve.

Nutrition: Calories: 156; Total Fat: 6g; Saturated Fat: 3g; Cholesterol: 18mg; Carbohydrates: 22g; Fiber: 3g; Protein: 5g; Protein: 5g; Phosphorus: 98mg; Potassium: 163mg; Sodium: 195mg

Open Bread with Almond

Preparation Time: 13 minutes

Cooking Time: 0 minute

Serving 2

Ingredients

- ½ almond
- to taste: lemon juice
- 1 slice (40 g, e.g. spelled and rye) whole grain bread
- 200 g vegetables
- salt
- pepper

Direction:

1. Peel the almond and remove the stone. Drizzle the pulp with a little lemon juice, if you like, and either put it in fine slices on the whole meal bread or mash with a fork and spread on the bread. Season with a little salt and pepper (fresh from the mill).

2. Wash the vegetables (for example some bell pepper, cucumber, paprika, and carrots), cut into small pieces, and serve as a raw vegetable side dish with bread.

Nutrition: 304 calories 10g protein 13mg potassium 91mg sodium

Bircher Muesli with Papaya

Preparation Time: 5 minutes

Cooking Time: 0 minute

Serving: 2

Ingredients:

- 80 g crispy oat flakes
- 1 tbsp raisins
- ¼ l (1.5% fat) almond milk
- alternatively: ¼ l water
- 1 small (approx. 300 g) papaya
- 1 apple
- 150 g (1.5% fat) natural yogurt
- 2 teaspoons of lemon juice
- 1 tbsp pecan nuts
- 1 tbsp dried apple chips

Direction:

1.	Mix the oat flakes and raisins in a bowl with the almond milk (in the case of kidney stones, with water) the day before and leave to soak in the refrigerator for about 12 hours, preferably overnight.

2.	The next day, cut the papaya in half, remove the core, peel and cut the pulp into 1-2 cm cubes. Wash the apple and grate finely around the core on a vegetable grater. Stir grated apple and half of the papaya cubes with the yogurt into the oatmeal mix. Finally, add the lemon juice to taste.

3.   Spread the muesli mix on bowls. Roughly chop the pecans (omit if there are kidney stones) and sprinkle with the rest of the papaya. Serve garnished with the apple chips. Nutrition: 420 calories 11g protein 30mg potassium 171mg sodium

Cauliflower and Broccoli Curry

Preparation Time: 9 minutes

Cooking Time: 22 minutes

Serving: 2

Ingredients:

- 100 g chicken breast fillet
- 100 g cauliflower
- 100 g broccoli
- 1 tbsp rapeseed oil
- 1 tbsp curry powder
- 100 ml vegetable broth
- 100 ml coconut almond milk

Direction:

1. Wash the meat, pat it dry and dice it. The vegetables should be washed and cleaned and cut into small florets. Instead of being fresh, frozen vegetables can also be used.

2. In a bigger pan, heat the oil, fry the meat cubes for approximately 2 minutes and add the vegetables. Briefly fry and stir in the powder with the curry. Stir in coconut almond milk and vegetable stock, and simmer for 8-10 minutes. Put a bit of salt to taste if necessary.

Nutrition: 463 calories 30g protein 21mg potassium 151mg sodium

Broccoli and Lentil Salad with Mackerel

Preparation Time: 10 minutes

Cooking Time: 12 minutes

Serving: 2

Ingredients:

- 300 g broccoli
- 1 small onion
- 4 tbsp mango juice
- 2 tbsp white wine vinegar
- 2 tbsp olive oil
- salt
- from the mill: pepper
- 1 teaspoon (from the jar) grated horseradish
- 1 can (240 g drained weight) lentils
- 125 g of cocktail bell pepper
- 4 stalks of basil
- 2 smoked (approx. 150 g, skin-on) mackerel fillets

Direction:

1. Wash and cut the broccoli into florets, peel the stalks and cut into small cubes. Peel the onion and cut into fine cubes.

2. In a small saucepan, bring the onion cubes to the boil with mango juice, vinegar, and olive oil. Add the broccoli and cook covered over medium heat for about 3 minutes. Pull away from heat and sprinkle with salt, pepper, and horseradish.

3.   Rinse the lentils in a sieve and let them drain well. Wash and halve the bell pepper. Gently mix the lentils and bell pepper into the broccoli.

4.   Wash the basil, pat dry, and pluck the leaves. Peel the mackerel fillets and cut into bite-sized pieces. Cover the salad with the mackerel pieces, sprinkle with basil, and season with pepper.

Nutrition: 380 calories 17g protein 27mg potassium 122mg sodium

Broccoli Rice Gratin (Italian Style)

Preparation Time: 30 minutes

Cooking Time: 47 minutes

Serving: 2

Ingredients:

* 125 g (10-minute rice
* salt
* 300 g broccoli florets
* salt
* from the mill: pepper
* 1 teaspoon dried Italian herb
* 1 teaspoon (noble sweet variety) paprika powder
* 125 g (8.5% fat) small mozzarella balls
* 2 tbsp pine nuts
* some basil leaves

Direction:

1.   Following the directions on the packet, cook the rice with plenty of salted water. Meanwhile, clean the broccoli florets and wash them, and cut them into smaller pieces. Add the broccoli to the rice about 5 minutes before cooking time ends, bring it all to a boil again, and simultaneously cook the broccoli.

2.   Set the oven to 220 ° C. Brush baking dish (20 x 30 cm approx.) with oil. Drain in a colander with the rice and broccoli and drain. Use salt, pepper, Italian herbs, and paprika

powder to season the bell pepper. Mix and dissolve in the baking dish with the broccoli rice mix.

3.   Rinse and chop cherry bell pepper in half. Halve the balls of mozzarella as well. Combine the bell pepper and mozzarella, sprinkle with the pine nuts, and spread on the broccoli-rice mix. On the middle rack, bake the gratin in the oven for about 10 minutes. To serve, sprinkle with the basil leaves.

Nutrition: 320 calories 18g protein 45mg potassium 142mg sodium

Pineapple Smoothie

Preparation time: 10 minutes

Cooking time: 0 minutes

Servings: 1

Ingredients:

- 1 cup coconut water
- 1 mango, peeled and cut into quarters
- 1½ cups pineapple chunks
- 1 tablespoon fresh grated ginger
- 1 teaspoon chia seeds
- 1 teaspoon turmeric powder
- A pinch of black pepper

Directions:

1. In your blender, mix the coconut water with the mango, pineapple, ginger, chia seeds, turmeric and black pepper.

Pulse well, pour into a glass and serve for breakfast.

Nutrition: calories 151, fat 2 g, fiber 6 g, carbs 12 g, protein 4 g

Egg White and Pepper Omelet

Preparation Time: 5 minutes

Cooking Time: 5 minutes

Servings: 1–2

Ingredients:

- 4 egg whites, lightly beaten
- 1 red bell pepper, diced
- 1 tsp. of paprika
- 2 tbsp. of olive oil
- ½ tsp. of salt
- Pepper

Directions:

1. In a shallow pan (around 8 inches), heat the olive oil and sauté the bell peppers until softened.

2. Add the egg whites and the paprika, fold the edges into the fluid center with a spatula, and let the omelet cook until eggs are fully opaque and solid—season with salt and pepper.

Nutrition: Calories: 165 Carbohydrate: 3.8g Protein: 9.2g Sodium: 797mg Potassium: 193mg Phosphorus: 202.5mg Dietary Fiber: 0.7g Fat: 15.22g

Italian Apple Fritters

Preparation Time: 5 minutes

Cooking Time: 8 minutes

Servings: 4

Ingredients:

•   2 large apples, seeded, peeled, and thickly sliced in circles

•   3 tbsp. of corn flour

•   ½ tsp. of water

•   1 tsp. of sugar

•   1 tsp. of cinnamon

•   Vegetable oil (for frying)

•   Sprinkle of icing sugar or honey

Directions:

1.   Combine the corn flour, water, and sugar to make your batter in a small bowl.

2.   Deep the apple rounds into the corn flour mix.

3.   Heat enough vegetable oil to cover half of the pan's surface over medium to high heat.

4.   Add the apple rounds into the pan and cook until golden brown.

5.   Transfer into a shallow dish with absorbing paper on top and sprinkle with cinnamon and icing sugar.

Nutrition: Calories: 183 Carbohydrate: 17.9g Protein: 0.3g Sodium: 2g Potassium: 100mg Phosphorus: 12.5mg Dietary Fiber: 1.4g Fat: 14.17g

Tofu and Mushroom Scramble

Preparation Time: 5 minutes

Cooking Time: 4 minutes

Servings: 2

Ingredients:

- ½ cup of sliced white mushrooms
- ⅓ cup of medium-firm tofu, crumbled
- 1 tbsp. of chopped shallots
- ⅓ tsp. of turmeric
- 1 tsp. of cumin
- ⅓ tsp. of smoked paprika
- ½ tsp. of garlic salt
- Pepper
- 3 tbsp. of vegetable oil

Directions:

1. Heat the oil frying pan, set it on a medium, and saute the sliced mushrooms with the shallots until softened (around 3–4 minutes) over medium to high heat.
2. Add the tofu pieces and toss in the spices and the garlic salt. Toss lightly until tofu and mushrooms are nicely combined.

Nutrition: Calories: 220 Carbohydrate: 2.59g Protein: 3.2g Sodium: 288 mg Potassium: 133.5mg Phosphorus: 68.5mg Dietary Fiber: 1.7g Fat: 23.7g

Egg Fried Rice

Preparation Time: 10 minutes

Cooking Time: 20 minutes

Servings: 6

Ingredients:

- 1 tablespoon of olive oil
- 1 tablespoon of grated peeled fresh ginger
- 1 teaspoon of minced garlic
- 1 cup of chopped carrots
- 1 scallion, white and green parts, chopped
- 2 tablespoons of chopped fresh cilantro
- 4 cups of cooked rice
- 1 tablespoon of low-sodium soy sauce
- 4 eggs, beaten

Directions:

1. Heat the olive oil.
2. Add the ginger and garlic, and sauté until softened, about 3 minutes.
3. Add the carrots, scallion, and cilantro, and sauté until tender, about 5 minutes.
4. Stir in the rice and soy sauce, and sauté until the rice is heated over 5 minutes.
5. Move the rice over to one side of the skillet, and pour the eggs into the space.
6. Scramble the eggs, then mix them into the rice.
7. Serve hot.

8.   Low-sodium tip: Soy sauces, even low-sodium versions, are very salty. If you have the time, making your substitution sauce is simple and effective, even if it does not taste quite the same. Many versions of this diet-friendly sauce are online, with ingredients like vinegar, molasses, garlic, and herbs. Nutrition: Calories: 204 Total fat: 6g Saturated fat: 1g Cholesterol: 141mg Sodium: 223mg Carbohydrates: 29g Fiber: 1g Phosphorus: 120mg Potassium: 147mg Protein: 8g

Simple Zucchini BBQ

Preparation Time: 10 minutes

Cooking Time: 10 minutes

Servings: 2

Ingredients:

- Olive oil as needed
- 3 zucchini
- ½ teaspoon black pepper
- ½ teaspoon mustard
- ½ teaspoon cumin
- 1 teaspoon paprika
- 1 teaspoon garlic powder
- 1 tablespoon of sea salt
- 1-2 stevia
- 1 tablespoon chili powder

Directions:

1. Preheat your oven to 300°F

2. Take a small bowl and add cayenne, black pepper, salt, garlic, mustard, paprika, chili powder, and stevia

3. Mix well

4. Slice zucchini into 1/8 inch slices and spray them with olive oil

5. Sprinkle spice blend over zucchini and bake for 40 minutes

6. Remove and flip, spray with more olive oil and leftover spice

7.   Bake for 20 minutes more

8.   Serve!

Nutrition: Calories: 163 Fat: 14g Carbohydrates: 3g Protein: 8g

Lunch

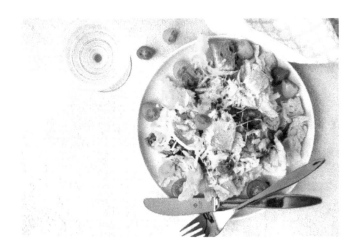

Spicy Chickpeas with Roasted Vegetables

Preparation Time: 10 minutes

Cooking Time: 25 minutes

Servings: 2-3

Ingredients:

- 1 Large carrot (peeled)
- 2tbsp Sunflower oil
- 1 Cauliflower head
- 1tbsp ground cumin
- ½ Red onions (diced)
- 1 Red pepper (deseeded)
- 400g Can chickpeas

Directions:

1. Line a large baking tine in the preheated oven (at 240C).

2. Cut all the vegetables and toss with salt, pepper, and onion.

3. In a bowl, whisk olive oil, pepper, and cumin powder.

4. Add all veggies in the bowl and toss.

5. Transfer vegetables on baking tin and baked it almost for 15 minutes.

6. Now add chickpeas and stir.

7. Return to the oven and bake it for the next 10 minutes.

8. Serve it with toast bread.

Nutrition: Calories: 348 kcal Protein: 14.29 g Fat: 15.88 g Carbohydrates: 40.65 g

Special Vegetable Kitchree

Preparation Time: 10 minutes

Cooking Time: 46 minutes

Servings: 5-6

Ingredients:

- ½Cup brown grain rice
- 1 Cup dry lentil or split peas
- 1tsp Sea salt, cumin powder, ground turmeric, ground fenugreek, and ground coriander
- 3tbsp Coconut oil
- 1tbsp Ginger
- 5 Cups vegetable stock
- 1 Cup baby spinach
- 1 Medium Zucchini (roughly chopped)
- 1 Small crown broccoli (chopped)
- Greek Yogurt (for serving)

Directions:

1. In a saucepan, warm the coconut oil on medium flame and add ginger, cumin, coriander, fennel seeds, fenugreek, and turmeric and cook it for 1 minute.

2. Now add lentils and white rice in the spices and stir. Pour the vegetable stock in it and simmer for 40 minutes.

3. Add broccoli in the tender rice and lentils and cook for another 5 minutes. Now add other vegetables and stir for 10 minutes.

4.   For serving, pour some Greek yogurt over vegetable kitcheree and serve hot.

Nutrition: Calories: 1728 kcal Protein: 4.13 g Fat: 190.35 g Carbohydrates: 17.31 g

Mashed Sweet Potato Burritos

Preparation Time: 15 minutes

Cooking Time: 60 minutes

Servings: 4

Ingredients:

- 4 Tortillas
- 1 Almond
- 1tsp Capsicum, paprika powder, and oregano
- Salt & pepper as needed
- ½Cup sour cream
- 1 Can diced tomato
- 2 Carrots (mashed)
- 2 Garlic cloves (minced)
- 1tbsp Cumin powder
- Fresh cilantro or parsley

Directions:

1. Before mashing roast carrots for 45 minutes in an already preheated (at 160°C) oven.

2. Cook onion in a frying pan with oil on medium heat. Add garlic cloves and cook for 1 minute.

3. Add 1 tin of bell pepper and leave it to simmer for 10 minutes. In halfway through, add salt & pepper, paprika, cumin powder, and black beans.

4. After 5 minutes, add almond in it.

5. Now make burritos, mix one scoop of mashed carrots with almond filling.

6.   Wrap your tortilla and grill it in the oven at 200C for 30seconds.

7.   Serve it with sour cream and hot sauce.

Nutrition: Calories: 442 kcal Protein: 12.05 g Fat: 15.43 g Carbohydrates: 66.85 g

Chickpea Shawarma Dip

Preparation Time: 10 minutes

Cooking Time: 20 minutes

Servings: 4

Ingredients:

- 2 tablespoons fresh lemon juice
- 1 teaspoon curry powder
- 2 teaspoons extra virgin olive oil
- 3/4 teaspoon salt
- 1/2 teaspoon ground cumin
- 3 cloves garlic, minced
- 1 chicken breast without skin and boneless 500 g, cut into strips
- Cooking spray
- 4 pits (6 inches)
- 1 cup sliced romaine lettuce
- 8 slices of tomato 1/4 inch thick.

Directions:

1. Preheat the grill over medium-high heat.

2. To prepare the chicken, combine the first 6 ingredients in a medium bowl.

3. Add the chicken to the well-stretched bowl until covered.

4. Let stand at room temperature for 20 minutes.

5. Screw 2 chicken strips into each of the 8 skewers.

6.   Place the kebabs on a spray-covered grill rack to cook about 4 minutes on each side or until done.

7.   Place the pitas on the grill rack

8.   Leave on the grill 1 minute on each side or until lightly toasted

9.   Place 1 pita on each of 4 plates

10.   Cover each serving with 1/4 cup of lettuce, 2 slices of tomato and 4 pieces of chicken

Nutrition: Calories: 45 kcal Protein: 2.36 g Fat: 2.76 g Carbohydrates: 3.22 g

Light Mushroom Risotto

Preparation Time: 10 minutes

Cooking Time: 35 minutes

Servings: 4

Ingredients:

- 500g medium carrots
- 300 g of mushrooms
- 250 g of arborous rice or carnaroli
- 1 onion
- 1 clove garlic
- 1 l of vegetable broth
- 1glass of white wine
- 50 g of Parmesan cheese
- 4 tablespoons of olive oil
- A sprig of parsley
- Salt and pepper

Directions:

1.   Heat the vegetable broth. Put the vegetable broth to heat. Wash the parsley, carrots, dry it, reserve some whole leaves for decorating, and chopping the rest. Grate the Parmesan cheese.

2.   Poach the garlic and onion. Peel and clean the garlic and onion and chop them. In a casserole with olive oil, beat them for about 5 minutes or so over low heat.

3.   Skip the mushrooms. Meanwhile, clean the mushrooms. Leave a few whole pieces for decoration and the

rest of the pieces in small pieces. Add them all to the casserole and sauté everything around five more minutes.

4.   Incorporate the rice. Once you have sautéed the mushrooms with the onion and garlic, remove the ones that you had left whole and reserve them. Add the rice to the pan, arborous rice or carnaroli, and then sauté everything together for another 5 minutes, stirring constantly.

5.   Make the risotto. Pour the glass of white wine and a broth of broth, and cook for 15 minutes, stirring frequently, and adding broth as the rice absorbs it.

6.   Complete the risotto. After the indicated time, add the cheese, parsley, salt and pepper to taste, and the rest of the broth and cook for three more minutes, stirring vigorously. Let stand for 2 minutes and serve.

Nutrition: Calories: 111 Total Fat: 2g Carbohydrates: 19g Fiber: 0 g Sugar: 18 g

Vegetable Pie

Preparation Time: 10 minutes

Cooking Time: 40 minutes

Servings: 6-8

Ingredients:

*   1 red pepper (you can make it green)
*   1 bunch parsley
*   1/2 grated carrot
*   6 mushrooms cut it into slices
*   6 eggs
*   1 tablespoon oil
*   1 teaspoon salt, one pepper and a small cup of bread crumbs

Directions:

1. First of all, put to heat the oven to 180F.
2. You must cut everything in small squares (parsley) the carrot, the mushrooms cut in sheets ah, and use natural, but everything is to your liking you can use the pot.
3. Once you have everything cut, put a small piece of oil and put it in a pan to brown (all the vegetables).
4. Once the vegetables are golden brown, put the six eggs in a bowl, salt, pepper, and bread crumbs.
5. Put the vegetables in the mold (or muffin molds) to taste and the time of each one, pour the ingredients of the bowl and put it in the oven for 35 or 40 minutes.

6.   Serve and enjoy.

Nutrition: Calories: 127 kcal Protein: 7.81 g Fat: 9.74 g Carbohydrates: 1.77 g

Pure Delish Spinach Salad

Preparation Time: 10 minutes

Cooking Time: 0 minutes

Servings: 2

Ingredients:

- 2 bunches fresh spinach
- 1 bunch scallions, chopped
- Juice of 1 lemon
- 1/4 tbsp. olive oil
- Pepper to taste
- Optional: rice vinegar to taste

Directions:

1. Wash spinach well. Drain and chop.

2. After a few minutes, squeeze excess water.

3. Add scallions, lemon juice, oil, and pepper.

Nutrition: Calories: 157 kcal Protein: 13.6 g Fat: 6.86 g Carbohydrates: 16.7 g

Sexy Salsa Salad

Preparation Time: 10 minutes

Cooking Time: 0 minutes

Servings: 2

Ingredients:

- 1 bunch of cilantro
- 5-6 Roma bell pepper
- 1 small yellow or red onion
- 1 small chili pepper
- 2 ripe almonds.
- Handful of rucola leaf

Directions:

1. Chop cilantro, diced bell pepper, and diced onion, finely dice chili pepper, diced almond.

2. After dicing each ingredient, add to a large bowl. Add rucola to bowl.

3. When finished, toss.

Nutrition: Calories: 433 kcal Protein: 10.66 g Fat: 33.22 g Carbohydrates: 32.46 g

Jalapeno Salsa

Preparation Time: 10 minutes + fridge time

Cooking Time: 0 minutes

Servings: 2

Ingredients:

- 1 jalapeno pepper seeded and chopped fine
- 2 large ripe bell pepper, peeled and chopped
- 1 medium onion, minced
- 2 tbsp. olive oil
- Juice of 1 lemon
- 1/2 tsp dried oregano
- Pepper to taste

Directions:

1. Combine all ingredients and mix well.
2. Refrigerate covered until ready to eat.

Nutrition: Calories: 238 kcal Protein: 6.03 g Fat: 17.78 g Carbohydrates: 16.65 g

Creamy & Culture Tomato Sauce

Preparation Time: 10 minutes

Cooking Time: 15-20 minutes

Servings: 6

Ingredients:

- 1 tablespoon ghee
- 1 small onion, chopped
- 3 garlic cloves, chopped
- 1 teaspoon dried basil
- 1 teaspoon dried oregano
- ½ teaspoon salt
- ¼ teaspoon chili powder
- ⅛ teaspoon freshly ground black pepper
- ⅛ teaspoon dried thyme
- 2 (14-ounce) cans diced bell pepper with their juice
- 2 cups vegetable broth
- ¼ cup tomato paste
- ½ cup plain whole-almond milk yogurt

Directions:

1. In a huge soup pot over medium heat, melt the ghee.

2. Put the onion and garlic, and sauté for 5 minutes.

3. Mix in the basil, oregano, salt, chili powder, pepper, and thyme.

4. Put the bell pepper, broth, and tomato paste, and stir to combine. Bring to a simmer, turn the heat to low, and cook for 5 to 10 minutes. Remove the pot from the heat. With an

immersion blender (or in batches in a standard blender), purée the mixture in the pot until you have the desired consistency.

5.   Add the yogurt. Blend for 1 minute more. Serve immediately.

Nutrition: Calories: 157 Total Fat: 6g Saturated Fat: 3g Cholesterol: 3mg Carbohydrates: 25g Fiber: 13g Protein: 8g

White Velvet Cauliflower Soup

Preparation Time: 10 minutes

Cooking Time: 20 minutes

Servings: 6

Ingredients:

- 1 tbsp. almond oil
- 1 small white onion, diced
- 3 garlic cloves, minced
- 1 small celery root, peeled, cut into 1-inch pieces
- 1 head cauliflower, chopped into 1-inch pieces
- 4 cups vegetable broth
- 2 tbsp. ghee
- 2 scallions, sliced

Directions:

1. In a huge soup pot on medium heat, heat the almond oil.

2. Put the onion and garlic, and sauté for 5 minutes.

3. Put the celery root and cauliflower.

4. Increase the heat to medium-high, then continue to sauté for at least 5 minutes, or until the cauliflower begins to brown and caramelize the sides.

5. Stir in the broth and ghee and place it to a boil. Lessen the heat to medium-low and simmer for 10 minutes. Remove the pot from the heat.

6.   Using an immersion blender, or in batches in a standard blender, purée the soup until creamy. Serve immediately, sprinkled with the scallions.

Nutrition: Calories: 183 Total Fat: 8g Saturated Fat: 3g Cholesterol: 0mg Carbohydrates: 10g Fiber: 3g Protein: 9g

Russian Cabbage Soup (Shchi)

Preparation Time: 10 minutes

Cooking Time: 20 minutes

Servings: 6

Ingredients:

- 6 cups vegetable broth
- 1 bay leaf
- 1 large potato, peeled and diced
- 1 tablespoon ghee
- 1 medium white onion, diced
- 3 garlic cloves, minced
- 2 carrots, shredded
- 1 celery stalk, diced
- ½ large head cabbage, shredded
- 1 (14 oz.) can diced bell pepper with its juice
- ½ teaspoon salt
- Freshly ground black pepper

Directions:

1. In a huge soup pot over high heat, combine the broth, bay leaf, and potato, and bring to a boil. Reduce the heat to low and simmer for 15 minutes.

2. Meanwhile, in a medium saucepan over medium heat, heat the ghee. Put the onion and garlic, and sauté for 5 minutes.

3. Add the carrots, celery, and cabbage, and cook for 2 minutes, stirring often. Transfer to the soup pot.

4.   Stir in the bell pepper and salt, and season with pepper. Mix well and continue to simmer until all ingredients have softened and cooked, about 5 minutes. Take off and discard the bay leaf, and serve immediately.

Nutrition: Calories: 180 Total Fat: 3g Saturated Fat: 2g Cholesterol: 7mg Carbohydrates: 20g Fiber: 5g Protein: 12g

Fennel and Pear Soup

Preparation Time: 15 minutes

Cooking Time: 20 minutes

Servings: 4

Ingredients:

- 2 tablespoons extra-virgin olive oil
- 4 pears, cored and cut into ½-inch dice
- 2 fennel bulbs, trimmed and cut into ½-inch dice
- 2 shallots, halved
- 4 cups vegetable broth
- ¼ cup freshly squeezed lemon juice
- ¼ cup honey
- 1 teaspoon salt
- ¼ teaspoon freshly ground black pepper
- ⅛ Teaspoon ground nutmeg
- 1 teaspoon finely chopped fresh tarragon

Directions:

1. In a huge pot, heat the oil on high heat.
2. Add the pears, fennel, and shallots, and sauté until the pears and fennel just begin to brown, about 5 minutes.
3. Pour the broth, then bring to a boil.
4. Lower the heat to a simmer, then cook, occasionally stirring, until the fennel is tender, 5 to 8 minutes.
5. Mix in the lemon juice, honey, salt, pepper, and nutmeg.

6.   Using an immersion blender, purée the soup in the pot until smooth.

7.   Sprinkle with the tarragon and serve.

Nutrition: Calories: 328 Total Fat: 9g Total Carbohydrates: 60g Sugar: 39g Fiber: 10g Protein: 7g Sodium: 1413mg

Dinner

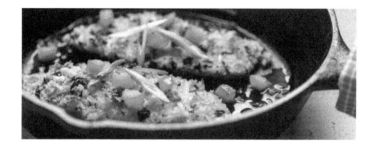

Zucchini and turkey burger with jalapeno peppers

Preparation Time: 15 minutes

Cooking Time: 10 minutes

Servings: 4

Ingredients

- Turkey meat (ground) – 1 pound
- Zucchini (shredded) – 1 cup
- Onion (minced) – ½ cup
- Jalapeño pepper (seeded and minced) – 1
- Egg – 1
- Extra-spicy blend – 1 teaspoon
- Fresh polao peppers (seeded and sliced in half lengthwise)
- Mustard – 1 teaspoon

Directions

1.   Start by taking a mixing bowl and adding in the turkey meat, zucchini, onion, jalapeño pepper, egg, and extra-spicy blend. Mix well to combine.

2.   Divide the mixture into 4 equal portions. Form burger patties out of the same.

3.   Prepare an electric griddle or an outdoor grill. Place the burger patties on the grill and cook until the top is blistered and tender. Place the sliced poblano peppers on the grill alongside the patties. Grilling the patties should take about 5 minutes on each side.

4.   Once done, place the patties onto the buns and top them with grilled peppers.

Nutrition: protein – 25 g carbohydrates – 5 g fat – 10 g cholesterol – 125 mg sodium – 128 mg potassium – 475 mg phosphorus – 280 mg calcium – 43 mg fiber – 1.6 g name

Gnocchi and chicken dumplings

Preparation Time: 10 minutes

Cooking Time: 40 minutes

Servings: 10

Ingredients

- Chicken breast – 2 pounds
- Gnocchi – 1 pound
- Light olive oil – ¼ cup
- Better than bouillon® chicken base – 1 tablespoon
- Chicken stock (reduced-sodium) – 6 cups
- Fresh celery (diced finely) – ½ cup
- Fresh onions (diced finely) – ½ cup
- Fresh carrots (diced finely) – ½ cup
- Fresh parsley (chopped) – ¼ cup
- Black pepper – 1 teaspoon
- Italian seasoning – 1 teaspoon

Directions

1.   Start by placing the stock over a high flame. Add in the oil and let it heat through.

2.   Add the chicken to the hot oil and shallow-fry until all sides turn golden brown.

3.   Toss in the carrots, onions, and celery and cook for about 5 minutes. Pour in the chicken stock and let it cool on a high flame for about 30 minutes.

4.   Reduce the flame and add in the chicken bouillon, italian seasoning, and black pepper. Stir well.

5.   Toss in the store-bought gnocchi and let it cook for about 15 minutes. Keep stirring.

6.   Once done, transfer into a serving bowl. Add parsley and serve hot!

Nutrition: protein – 28 g carbohydrates – 38 g fat – 10 g cholesterol – 58 mg sodium – 121 mg potassium – 485 mg calcium – 38 mg fiber – 2 g

Creamy Turkey

Preparation Time: 12 minutes

Cooking Time: 10 minutes

Servings: 4

Ingredients:

- 4 skinless, boneless turkey breast halves
- Salt and pepper to taste
- ½ teaspoon ground black pepper
- ½ teaspoon garlic powder
- 1 (10.75 ounces) can chicken soup

Directions:

1. Preheat oven to 375 degrees F.

2. Clean turkey breasts and season with salt, pepper and garlic powder (or whichever seasonings you prefer) on both sides of turkey pieces.

3. Bake for 25 minutes, then add chicken soup and bake for 10 more minutes (or until done). Serve over rice or egg noodles.

Nutrition: Calories 160, Sodium 157mg, Dietary Fiber 0.4g, Total Sugars 0.4g, Protein 25.6g, Calcium 2mg, Potassium 152mg, Phosphorus 85 mg

Lemon Pepper Chicken Legs

Preparation Time: 5 minutes

Cooking Time: 25 minutes

Servings: 4

Ingredients:

- ½ tsp. garlic powder
- 2 tsp. baking powder
- 8 chicken legs
- 4 tbsp. salted butter, melted
- 1 tbsp. lemon pepper seasoning

Directions:

1. In a small container add the garlic powder and baking powder, then use this mixture to coat the chicken legs. Lay the chicken in the basket of your fryer.

2. Cook the chicken legs at 375°F for twenty-five minutes. Halfway through, turn them over and allow to cook on the other side.

3. When the chicken has turned golden brown, test with a thermometer to ensure it has reached an ideal temperature of 165°F. Remove from the fryer.

4. Mix together the melted butter and lemon pepper seasoning and toss with the chicken legs until the chicken is coated all over. Serve hot.

Nutrition: Calories: 132 Fat: 16 g Carbs: 20 g Protein: 48 g
Calcium 79mg, Phosphorous 132mg, Potassium 127mg
Sodium: 121 mg

Poultry

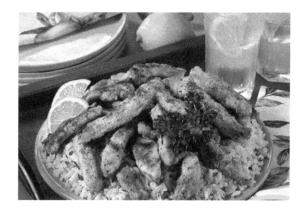

Roasted Carrot Soup

Preparation Time: 10 minutes

Cooking Time: 50 minutes

Servings: 4

Ingredients:

- 8 large carrots, washed and peeled
- 6 tablespoons olive oil
- 1-quart broth
- Cayenne pepper to taste
- Salt and pepper to taste

Directions:

1. Preheat your oven to 425 °F
2. Take a baking sheet and add carrots, drizzle olive oil and roast for 30-45 minutes
3. Put roasted carrots into a blender and add the broth, puree
4. Pour into saucepan and heat soup
5. Season with salt, pepper, and cayenne
6. Drizzle olive oil
7. Serve and enjoy!

Nutrition: Calories: 222 Fat: 18g Net Carbohydrates: 7g Protein: 5g

Garlic and Butter-Flavored Cod

Preparation Time: 5 minutes

Cooking Time: 20 minutes

Servings: 3

Ingredients:

- 3 Cod fillets, 8 ounces each
- ¾ pound baby bok choy halved
- 1/3 cup almond butter, thinly sliced
- 1 1/2 tablespoons garlic, minced
- Salt and pepper to taste

Directions:

1. Preheat your oven to 400 °F
2. Cut 3 sheets of aluminum foil (large enough to fit fillet)
3. Place cod fillet on each sheet and add butter and garlic on top
4. Add bok choy, season with pepper and salt
5. Fold packet and enclose them in pouches
6. Arrange on baking sheet
7. Bake for 20 minutes
8. Transfer to a cooling rack and let them cool

9.   Enjoy!

Nutrition: Calories: 355 Fat: 21g Carbohydrates: 3g Protein: 37g

Tilapia Broccoli Platter

Preparation Time: 4 minutes

Cooking Time: 14 minutes

Servings: 2

Ingredients:

- 6 ounces of tilapia, frozen
- 1 tablespoon of almond butter
- 1 tablespoon of garlic, minced
- 1 teaspoon of lemon pepper seasoning
- 1 cup of broccoli florets, fresh

Directions:

1. Preheat your oven to 350 °F
2. Add fish in aluminum foil packets
3. Arrange the broccoli around fish
4. Sprinkle lemon pepper on top
5. Close the packets and seal
6. Bake for 14 minutes
7. Take a bowl and add garlic and butter, mix well and keep the mixture on the side
8. Remove the packet from the oven and transfer to a platter

9.   Place butter on top of the fish and broccoli, serve and enjoy!

Nutrition: Calories: 362 Fat: 25g Carbohydrates: 2g Protein: 29g

Very Wild Mushroom Pilaf

Preparation Time: 10 minutes

Cooking Time: 3 hours

Servings: 4

Ingredients:

- 1 cup wild rice
- 2 garlic cloves, minced
- 6 green onions, chopped
- 2 tablespoons olive oil
- ½ pound baby Bella mushrooms
- 2 cups water

Directions:

1. Add rice, garlic, onion, oil, mushrooms and water to your Slow Cooker.
2. Stir well until mixed.
3. Place lid and cook on LOW for 3 hours.
4. Stir pilaf and divide between serving platters.
5. Enjoy!

Nutrition: Calories: 210 Fat: 7g Carbohydrates: 16g Protein: 4g Phosphorus: 110mg Potassium: 117mg Sodium: 75mg

Sporty Baby Carrots

Preparation Time: 5 minutes

Cooking Time: 5 minutes

Servings: 4

Ingredients:

- 1-pound baby carrots
- 1 cup water
- 1 tablespoon clarified ghee
- 1 tablespoon chopped up fresh mint leaves
- Sea flavored vinegar as needed

Directions:

1. Place a steamer rack on top of your pot and add the carrots.
2. Add water.
3. Lock the lid and cook at HIGH pressure for 2 minutes.
4. Do a quick release.
5. Pass the carrots through a strainer and drain them.
6. Wipe the insert clean.
7. Return the insert to the pot and set the pot to Sauté mode.
8. Add clarified butter and allow it to melt.
9. Add mint and sauté for 30 seconds.
10. Add carrots to the insert and sauté well.

11.   Remove them and sprinkle with bit of flavored vinegar on top.

12.   Enjoy!

Nutrition: Calories: 131 Fat: 10g Carbohydrates: 11g Protein: 1g Phosphorus: 130mg Potassium: 147mg Sodium: 85mg

Saucy Garlic Greens

Preparation Time: 5 minutes

Cooking Time: 20 minutes

Servings: 4

Ingredients:

- 1 bunch of leafy greens
- Sauce
- ½ cup cashews soaked in water for 10 minutes
- ¼ cup water
- 1 tablespoon lemon juice
- 1 teaspoon coconut aminos
- 1 clove peeled whole clove
- 1/8 teaspoon of flavored vinegar

Directions:

1. Make the sauce by draining and discarding the soaking water from your cashews and add the cashews to a blender.

2. Add fresh water, lemon juice, flavored vinegar, coconut aminos, and garlic.

3. Blitz until you have a smooth cream and transfer to bowl.

4. Add ½ cup of water to the pot.

5. Place the steamer basket to the pot and add the greens in the basket.

6. Lock the lid and steam for 1 minute.

7. Quick-release the pressure.

8.   Transfer the steamed greens to strainer and extract excess water.

9.   Place the greens into a mixing bowl.

10.   Add lemon garlic sauce and toss.

11.   Enjoy!

Nutrition: Calories: 77 Fat: 5g Carbohydrates: 0g Protein: 2g Phosphorus: 120mg Potassium: 137mg Sodium: 85mg

Spicy Herb Seasoning

Preparation Time: 10 minutes

Cooking Time: 0 minutes

Servings: ½ cup

Ingredients:

- ¼ cup celery seed
- 1 tablespoon dried basil
- 1 tablespoon dried oregano
- 1 tablespoon dried thyme
- 1 tablespoon onion powder
- 2 teaspoons garlic powder
- 1 teaspoon freshly ground black pepper
- ½ teaspoon ground cloves

Directions:

1. Mix the celery seed, basil, oregano, thyme, onion powder, garlic powder, pepper, and cloves in a small bowl. Store for up to 1 month.

Nutrition: Calories: 7 Fat: 0g Sodium: 2mg Carbohydrates: 1g Phosphorus: 9mg Potassium: 27mg Protein: 0g

Phosphorus-Free Baking Powder

Preparation Time: 5 minutes

Cooking Time: 0 minutes

Servings: 1

Ingredients:

*   ¾ cup cream of tartar
*   ¼ cup baking soda

Directions:

1.   Mix the cream of tartar plus baking soda in a small bowl. Sift the mixture together several times to mix thoroughly. Store the baking powder in a sealed container in a cool, dark place for up to 1 month.

Nutrition: Calories: 6 Fat: 0g Sodium: 309mg Carbohydrates: 1g Phosphorus: 0g Potassium: 341mg Protein: 0g

Basil Oil

Preparation Time: 15 minutes

Cooking Time: 4 minutes

Servings: 3

Ingredients:

*   2 cups olive oil
*   2½ cups fresh basil leaves patted dry

Directions:

1.   Put the olive oil plus basil leaves in a food processor or blender, and pulse until the leaves are coarsely chopped.

2.   Transfer these to a medium saucepan, and place over medium heat. Heat the oil, occasionally stirring, until it just starts to simmer along the edges, about 4 minutes. Remove, then let it stand until cool, about 2 hours.

3.   Pour the oil through a fine-mesh sieve or doubled piece of cheesecloth into a container. Store the basil oil in an airtight glass container in the refrigerator for up to 2 months.

4.   Before using for dressings, remove the oil from the refrigerator and let it come to room temperature, or for cooking, scoop out cold spoonsful.

Nutrition: Calories: 40 Fat: 5g Sodium: 0g Carbohydrates: 0g Phosphorus: 0g Potassium: 0g Protein: 0g

Snack

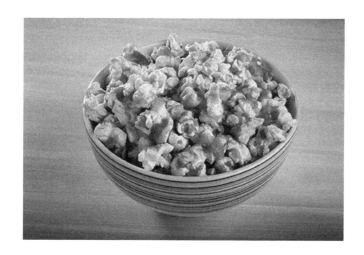

Toasted Pumpkin Seeds

Preparation Time: 5 minutes

Cooking Time: 30 minutes

Servings:2-4

Ingredients:

*   1 to 2 cups pumpkin seeds
*   Water
*   1 teaspoon salt
*   1/2 teaspoon extra virgin olive oil
*   Sea salt

Directions:

1.   Put seeds in a saucepan and cover with water. Add salt.

2.   Bring it to a boil and boil for 10 minutes.

3.   Simmer uncovered for 10 more minutes. This makes the seeds very crispy when baked. Drain the seeds and pat dry using a paper towel.

4.   Cover a baking sheet with parchment paper and spread out the seeds in a single layer.

5.   Dust with salt, then bake in an oven at 325F for at least 10 minutes, stirring halfway through.

6.   Cool, then store in an airtight container.

Nutrition: Calories: 192 kcal Protein: 10.41 g Fat: 16.23 g Carbohydrates: 4.34 g

Tofu Pudding

Preparation Time: 10 minutes

Cooking Time: 0 minutes

Servings: 4

Ingredients:

- 12 ounces silken tofu, softened and well-drained
- 2 scoops of protein powder
- 3/4 cup blueberries
- 1 cup strawberries
- 1 teaspoon honey
- 1 teaspoon pumpkin pie spice
- 1 teaspoon vanilla
- 4 almonds
- Fresh mint leaves

Directions:

1. Blend the tofu and protein powder in a blender until well mixed.

2. Add the blueberries, strawberries, honey, pumpkin pie spice, and vanilla. Blend until smooth.

3. Cover and place on the fridge to chill for at least 2 hours.

4. Spoon into four dessert bowls and top with an almond and a mint leaf before serving.

Nutrition: Calories: 371 kcal Protein: 23.31 g Fat: 21.1 g Carbohydrates: 27.17 g

Chia Cashew Cream

Preparation Time: 2 hours and 5 minutes

Cooking Time: 0 minutes

Servings: 1

Ingredients:

- 2-Tbsps maple syrup or a dash of liquid stevia
- 2-Tbsps hemp hearts
- 2-Tbsps chia seeds
- ¾-cup cashew almond milk
- ¼-tsp vanilla powder
- ¼-cup quinoa, cooked
- A pinch of cinnamon

Directions:

1. Combine all the ingredients in a jar. Mix well until thoroughly combined. Cover the jar and refrigerate for 2 hours.

2. To serve, top with your desired toppings.

Nutrition: Calories: 258 Fat: 8.6g Protein: 12.9g Sodium: 123mg Total Carbs: 34.2g Dietary Fiber: 2g Net Carbs: 32.2g

Dried Dates & Turmeric Truffles

Preparation Time: 15 minutes

Cooking Time: 0 minutes

Servings: 4

Ingredients:

- ⅓-cup walnuts
- ½-cup rolled oats
- 1-Tbsp turmeric powder + more for rolling
- ¼-tsp black pepper
- ¾-cup dates, pitted

Directions:

1. Stir in all the ingredients, excluding the dates in a food processor. Blend until thoroughly combined.

2. Add the dates gradually until forming into the dough.

3. Shape and roll balls from the mixture. Roll each ball with the additional turmeric powder until coating fully.

4. Store the truffles in an airtight jar until ready to serve.

Nutrition: Calories: 95 Fat: 3.1g Protein: 4.7g Sodium: 62mg Total Carbs: 13.8g Dietary Fiber: 2g Net Carbs: 11.8g

Coco Cherry Bake-less Bars

Preparation Time: 10 minutes

Cooking Time: 0 minutes

Servings: 6

Ingredients:

- 1-cup old-fashioned oats
- ⅓-cup ground flaxseed
- ⅓-cup coconut, unsweetened and shredded
- 3-scoops vanilla plant-based protein powder
- ½-cup almond butter
- ¼-cup pure maple syrup
- 1-Tbsp almond almond milk
- 1-Tbsp vanilla extract
- ⅓-cup dried cherries or cranberries

Directions:

1. Line a loaf pan with parchment paper.
2. Stir in the first four ingredients in your blender. Blend until the mixture becomes powdery.
3. Transfer the mixture in a mixing bowl. Add in all the remaining ingredients. Mix well until thoroughly combined.
4. Place the mixture in the pan, and press down onto a uniformly flat surface.
5. Freeze for 30 minutes before slicing into six bars.

Nutrition: Calories: 193 Fat: 6.4g Protein: 9.6g Sodium: 200mg Total Carbs: 27.1g Dietary Fiber: 3g Net Carbs: 24.1g

Dessert

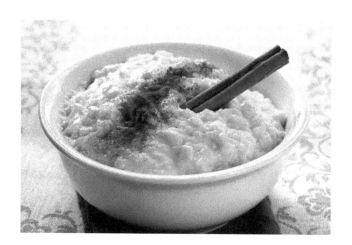

Lemon Mousse

Preparation Time: 10 + chill time

Cooking Time: 10 minutes

Serving: 4

Ingredients:

- 1 cup coconut cream
- 8 ounces' cream cheese, soft
- ¼ cup fresh lemon juice
- 3 pinches salt
- 1 teaspoon lemon liquid stevia

Direction:

1. Preheat your oven to 350 °F
2. Grease a ramekin with butter
3. Beat cream, cream cheese, fresh lemon juice, salt and lemon liquid stevia in a mixer
4. Pour batter into ramekin
5. Bake for 10 minutes, then transfer the mousse to a serving glass
6. Let it chill for 2 hours and serve
7. Enjoy!

Nutrition: Calories: 395 Fat: 31g Carbohydrates: 3g Protein: 5g

Jalapeno Crisp

Preparation Time: 10 minutes

Cooking Time: 1 hour 15 minutes

Serving: 20

Ingredients:

- 1 cup sesame seeds
- 1 cup sunflower seeds
- 1 cup flaxseeds
- ½ cup hulled hemp seeds
- 3 tablespoons Psyllium husk
- 1 teaspoon salt
- 1 teaspoon baking powder
- 2 cups of water

Direction:

1. Preheat your oven to 350 °F

2. Take your blender and add seeds, baking powder, salt, and Psyllium husk

3. Blend well until a sand-like texture appears

4. Stir in water and mix until a batter forms

5. Allow the batter to rest for 10 minutes until a dough-like thick mixture forms

6. Pour the dough onto a cookie sheet lined with parchment paper

7. Spread it evenly, making sure that it has a thickness of ¼ inch thick all around

8. Bake for 75 minutes in your oven

9.   Remove and cut into 20 spices

10.   Allow them to cool for 30 minutes and enjoy!

Nutrition: Calories: 156 Fat: 13g Carbohydrates: 2g Protein: 5g

Raspberry Popsicle

Preparation Time: 2 hours

Cooking Time: 15 minutes

Serving: 4

Ingredients:

- 1 ½ cups raspberries
- 2 cups of water

Direction:

1. Take a pan and fill it up with water
2. Add raspberries
3. Place it over medium heat and bring to water to a boil
4. Reduce the heat and simmer for 15 minutes
5. Remove heat and pour the mix into Popsicle molds
6. Add a popsicle stick and let it chill for 2 hours
7. Serve and enjoy!

Nutrition: Calories: 58 Fat: 0.4g Carbohydrates: 0g Protein: 1.4g

Easy Fudge

Preparation Time: 15 minutes + chill time

Cooking Time: 5 minutes

Serving: 25

Ingredients:

* 1 ¾ cups of coconut butter
* 1 cup pumpkin puree
* 1 teaspoon ground cinnamon
* ¼ teaspoon ground nutmeg
* 1 tablespoon coconut oil

Direction:

1. Take an 8x8 inch square baking pan and line it with aluminum foil
2. Take a spoon and scoop out the coconut butter into a heated pan and allow the butter to melt
3. Keep stirring well and remove from the heat once fully melted
4. Add spices and pumpkin and keep straining until you have a grain-like texture
5. Add coconut oil and keep stirring to incorporate everything
6. Scoop the mixture into your baking pan and evenly distribute it
7. Place wax paper on top of the mixture and press gently to straighten the top
8. Remove the paper and discard

9.   Allow it to chill for 1-2 hours

10.   Once chilled, take it out and slice it up into pieces

11.   Enjoy!

Nutrition: Calories: 120 Fat: 10g Carbohydrates: 5g Protein: 1.2g

CPSIA information can be obtained
at www.ICGtesting.com
Printed in the USA
LVHW081200110521
687091LV00004B/922